BRAIN CANCER COOKBOOK

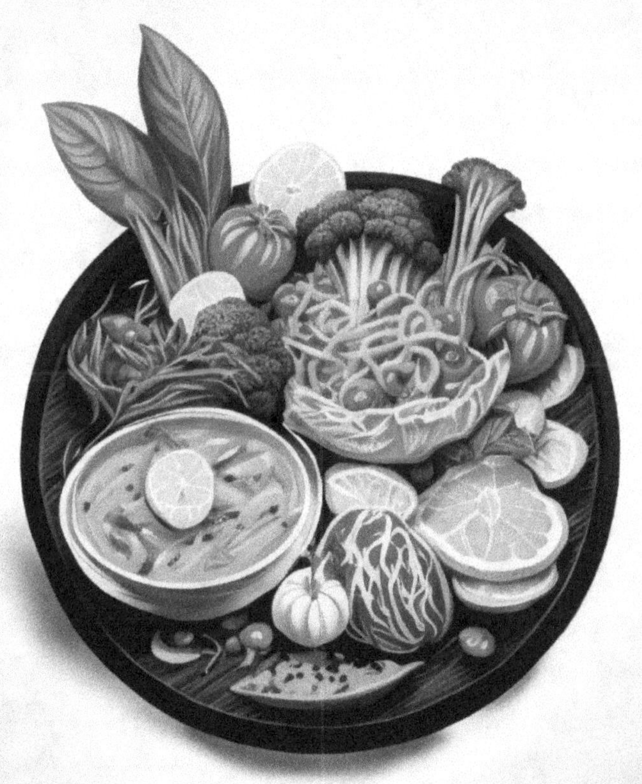

GET READY, LET'S FIGHT!

THIS BOOK BELONGS TO

Brain Cancer Cookbook

==================================

Feeding Hope, Nurturing Health

Jetta Harlow Olson

Attribution: The resources utilized to design this cover were obtained from pexels.com.

ISBN: 9798857270813

Imprint: Independently Published

Disclaimer

This book's instructions, recommendations, or methods are not intended to replace professional medical guidance, diagnosis, or care. The information in this book is only meant to be used for educational purposes; it should not be used as a replacement for professional medical advice from a healthcare provider.

The authors and publisher of this book disclaim any responsibility for any negative effects or outcomes attributable to the use of the knowledge, suggestions, or methods offered in this book. Readers should speak with their doctor before beginning any new health or wellness program.

Despite the fact that the knowledge and research upon which the information in this book is based is up-to-date, medical procedures and recommendations may alter over time.

It is advised that readers seek out additional information and keep current with healthcare trends.

The authors' views are the only ones that are expressed in this book; they do not necessarily represent the publisher's views. The authors and publisher do not endorse or recommend any companies, items, or services that are mentioned in this book.

Despite making every effort to ensure the accuracy and comprehensiveness of the information in this book, the authors and publisher make no promises or representations of any kind, either explicitly or implicitly, regarding the information's suitability, reliability, or availability.

Any risks associated with relying on the information in this book are assumed by the reader.

Contents

1. Personal Motivation for the Cookbook

Creating a Brain Cancer Cookbook is a deeply personal and meaningful endeavor that's driven by my passion for helping those affected by this challenging condition. My motivation comes from a desire to provide nourishment, comfort, and support to individuals and their loved ones on their journey through brain cancer treatment and recovery.

Witnessing the struggles faced by those with brain cancer has ignited my commitment to making a positive impact. This cookbook is my way of extending a helping hand, offering a source of inspiration, and promoting well-being through nutrition during a time when maintaining health is of utmost importance.

I understand the importance of providing recipes that are not only delicious but also tailored to the unique dietary needs of brain cancer patients. My motivation comes from a heartfelt wish to make their culinary experience enjoyable, nourishing, and uplifting. Every recipe is crafted with care, keeping in mind the nutritional requirements that can aid in managing symptoms, boosting immunity, and enhancing overall quality of life.

Through this cookbook, I aspire to instill a sense of hope and resilience in those affected by brain cancer. I believe that a well-balanced and nourishing diet can serve as a beacon of positivity amidst challenging times. My ultimate goal is to create a collection of recipes that not only provide sustenance but also contribute to the holistic well-being of individuals and their support networks.

This cookbook represents my commitment to making a difference and supporting those facing brain cancer with love, empathy, and a genuine dedication to their health and happiness.

Important Note: These recipes offer a variety of nutrient-rich ingredients and cater to different dietary preferences. Remember to tailor the portion sizes and ingredients to suit individual needs and dietary restrictions. Always consult with a healthcare professional before making significant changes to a patient's diet, especially for individuals undergoing cancer treatment.

2. Creamy Oatmeal with Berries

Ingredients:

- 1/2 cup rolled oats

- 1 cup milk (dairy or plant-based)

- 1/2 cup mixed berries (blueberries, strawberries, raspberries)

- 1 tablespoon honey or maple syrup (optional)

- 1 tablespoon chopped nuts (almonds, walnuts)

Instructions:

1. Combine oats and milk in a microwave-safe bowl.

2. Microwave on high for 2-3 minutes, stirring occasionally.

3. Top with mixed berries, honey or maple syrup, and chopped nuts.

3. Lentil and Vegetable Soup

Ingredients:

- 1 cup dried lentils (rinsed and drained)
- 4 cups low-sodium vegetable broth
- 1 cup diced carrots
- 1 cup diced celery
- 1 cup diced zucchini
- 1 cup diced tomatoes
- 1 teaspoon dried thyme
- Salt and pepper to taste

Instructions:

1. In a large pot, combine lentils, broth, carrots, celery, zucchini, tomatoes, and thyme.
2. Bring to a boil, then reduce heat and simmer for 20-25 minutes until lentils are tender.
3. Season with salt and pepper before serving.

4. Baked Salmon with Quinoa and Roasted Vegetables

Ingredients:

- 2 salmon fillets

- 1 cup quinoa

- 2 cups mixed vegetables (bell peppers, broccoli, asparagus)

- 2 tablespoons olive oil

- Lemon juice

- Fresh herbs (such as parsley or dill)

- Salt and pepper to taste

Instructions:

1. Preheat the oven to 375°F (190°C).

2. Place salmon fillets on a baking sheet and drizzle with lemon juice, olive oil, salt, and pepper. Bake for 15-20 minutes or until cooked through.

3. While the salmon is baking, cook quinoa according to package instructions.

4. Toss mixed vegetables with olive oil, salt, and pepper. Roast in the oven for 15-20 minutes.

5. Serve salmon over cooked quinoa, accompanied by roasted vegetables. Garnish with fresh herbs.

5. Soft Tofu and Vegetable Stir-Fry

Ingredients:

- 1 block soft tofu, cubed
- 2 cups mixed stir-fry vegetables (bell peppers, snap peas, carrots)
- 2 tablespoons low-sodium soy sauce
- 1 tablespoon sesame oil
- 1 teaspoon minced ginger
- 1 teaspoon minced garlic
- 2 green onions, sliced
- 1 tablespoon sesame seeds

Instructions:

1. In a wok or skillet, heat sesame oil over medium-high heat. Add ginger and garlic, sauté for 1-2 minutes.

2. Add tofu and stir-fry vegetables. Cook until vegetables are tender-crisp.

3. Drizzle with soy sauce and toss to combine.

4. Serve over brown rice or whole-grain noodles, garnished with sliced green onions and sesame seeds.

6. Fruit and Yogurt Parfait

Ingredients:

- 1 cup plain Greek yogurt
- 1 cup mixed fresh fruits (berries, kiwi, mango)
- 2 tablespoons granola
- 1 tablespoon honey

Instructions:

1. In a glass or bowl, layer Greek yogurt, mixed fruits, and granola.
2. Drizzle with honey before serving.

7. Spinach and Mushroom Egg Scramble

Ingredients:

- 3 eggs
- 1 cup fresh spinach, chopped
- 1/2 cup mushrooms, sliced
- 1/4 cup diced onions
- 1/4 cup shredded low-fat cheese (optional)
- Salt and pepper to taste
- 1 teaspoon olive oil

Instructions:

1. Heat olive oil in a non-stick skillet over medium heat.
2. Add onions and mushrooms, sauté until tender.
3. Whisk eggs in a bowl and pour into the skillet.
4. Add chopped spinach and cook, stirring gently until eggs are scrambled and cooked.
5. Season with salt and pepper, and sprinkle cheese on top if desired.

8. Quinoa and Black Bean Salad:

Ingredients:

- 1 cup cooked quinoa
- 1 cup canned black beans, rinsed and drained
- 1 cup diced cucumber
- 1 cup diced red bell pepper
- 1/4 cup chopped fresh cilantro
- 2 tablespoons lime juice
- 2 tablespoons olive oil
- Salt and pepper to taste

Instructions:

1. In a large bowl, combine cooked quinoa, black beans, cucumber, bell pepper, and cilantro.

2. In a separate bowl, whisk together lime juice, olive oil, salt, and pepper.

3. Drizzle the dressing over the quinoa mixture and toss to combine.

9. Chicken and Vegetable Stir-Fry

Ingredients:

- 1 boneless, skinless chicken breast, thinly sliced
- 2 cups mixed stir-fry vegetables (broccoli, bell peppers, carrots)
- 2 tablespoons low-sodium soy sauce
- 1 tablespoon hoisin sauce
- 1 teaspoon minced ginger
- 1 teaspoon minced garlic
- 1 tablespoon vegetable oil

Instructions:

1. In a wok or skillet, heat vegetable oil over medium-high heat.
2. Add ginger and garlic, sauté for 1-2 minutes.
3. Add sliced chicken and cook until no longer pink.
4. Add mixed vegetables and stir-fry until tender.
5. Mix in soy sauce and hoisin sauce. Cook for an additional minute.
6. Serve over brown rice or whole-grain noodles.

10.Roasted Sweet Potato and Kale Salad

Ingredients:

- 2 cups diced sweet potatoes
- 4 cups chopped kale leaves
- 1/4 cup dried cranberries
- 1/4 cup chopped walnuts
- 2 tablespoons olive oil
- 2 tablespoons balsamic vinegar
- Salt and pepper to taste

Instructions:

1. Preheat the oven to 400°F (200°C).

2. Toss diced sweet potatoes with 1 tablespoon olive oil, salt, and pepper. Roast for 20-25 minutes or until tender.

3. In a large bowl, massage kale leaves with remaining olive oil and balsamic vinegar.

4. Add roasted sweet potatoes, dried cranberries, and chopped walnuts to the bowl. Toss to combine.

11.Berry Smoothie Bowl

Ingredients:

- 1 cup mixed berries (strawberries, blueberries, raspberries)

- 1 banana

- 1/2 cup plain Greek yogurt

- 1/4 cup almond milk (or milk of choice)

- 2 tablespoons granola

- 1 tablespoon chia seeds

Instructions:

1. Blend mixed berries, banana, Greek yogurt, and almond milk until smooth.

2. Pour the smoothie into a bowl.

3. Top with granola and chia seeds.

12.Mashed Cauliflower with Herbs

Ingredients:

- 1 medium head of cauliflower, cut into florets
- 2 tablespoons unsalted butter or olive oil
- 1/4 cup fresh herbs (parsley, chives, thyme), chopped
- Salt and pepper to taste

Instructions:

1. Steam or boil cauliflower florets until tender.
2. Drain and transfer to a bowl. Mash with a potato masher or fork.
3. Mix in butter or olive oil, fresh herbs, salt, and pepper.

13. Baked Chicken and Vegetable Casserole

Ingredients:

- 2 boneless, skinless chicken breasts, cubed
- 2 cups mixed vegetables (carrots, green beans, peas)
- 1 cup diced potatoes
- 1/2 cup low-sodium chicken broth
- 2 tablespoons olive oil
- 1 teaspoon dried rosemary
- Salt and pepper to taste

Instructions:

1. Preheat the oven to 375°F (190°C).

2. In a baking dish, combine chicken, mixed vegetables, and diced potatoes.

3. Drizzle with olive oil and chicken broth. Sprinkle with dried rosemary, salt, and pepper.

4. Cover with aluminum foil and bake for 30 minutes. Remove foil and bake for an additional 15 minutes or until chicken is cooked and vegetables are tender.

14.Cottage Cheese and Fruit Parfait

Ingredients:

- 1 cup low-fat cottage cheese
- 1 cup mixed fresh fruits (pineapple, kiwi, grapes)
- 2 tablespoons chopped nuts (pecans, almonds)
- 1 tablespoon honey

Instructions:

1. In a glass or bowl, layer cottage cheese and mixed fruits.
2. Sprinkle with chopped nuts and drizzle with honey.

15.Vegetable and Rice Stuffed Bell Peppers

Ingredients:

- 4 bell peppers, tops removed and seeds removed

- 1 cup cooked brown rice

- 1 cup mixed vegetables (corn, peas, carrots)

- 1/2 cup diced tomatoes

- 1/4 cup shredded low-fat cheese (optional)

- 1 teaspoon dried oregano

- Salt and pepper to taste

Instructions:

1. Preheat the oven to 350°F (175°C).

2. In a bowl, mix cooked brown rice, mixed vegetables, diced tomatoes, dried oregano, salt, and pepper.

3. Stuff the bell peppers with the rice and vegetable mixture.

4. Place stuffed peppers in a baking dish. If desired, sprinkle shredded cheese on top.

5. Bake for 25-30 minutes or until the peppers are tender.

16. Coconut Chia Pudding with Mango

Ingredients:

- 1/4 cup chia seeds

- 1 cup coconut milk (canned or carton)

- 1 tablespoon honey or maple syrup

- 1 ripe mango, diced

Instructions:

1. In a bowl, combine chia seeds, coconut milk, and honey or maple syrup. Stir well.

2. Refrigerate for at least 2 hours or overnight, stirring occasionally to prevent clumps.

3. Serve the chia pudding with diced mango on top.

17.Creamy Broccoli and Potato Soup

Ingredients:

- 2 cups broccoli florets

- 2 medium potatoes, peeled and diced

- 1 small onion, chopped

- 2 cups low-sodium vegetable broth

- 1 cup milk (dairy or plant-based)

- 1 tablespoon olive oil

- Salt and pepper to taste

Instructions:

1. In a large pot, heat olive oil over medium heat. Add chopped onion and sauté until translucent.

2. Add diced potatoes and broccoli florets, then pour in the vegetable broth. Simmer until vegetables are tender.

3. Use an immersion blender to blend the soup until smooth.

4. Stir in milk, and season with salt and pepper. Heat gently before serving.

18.Turkey and Cranberry Wrap

Ingredients:

- 4 whole wheat tortillas
- 1 cup cooked and thinly sliced turkey breast
- 1/2 cup baby spinach leaves
- 1/4 cup cranberry sauce
- 1/4 cup crumbled feta cheese (optional)

Instructions:

1. Lay out the tortillas and divide the turkey slices among them.

2. Top each with baby spinach, cranberry sauce, and crumbled feta.

3. Roll up the tortillas, tucking in the sides as you go. Slice in half and serve.

19. Herbed Quinoa Stuffed Bell Peppers

Ingredients:

- 4 bell peppers, tops removed and seeds removed
- 1 cup cooked quinoa
- 1/2 cup diced tomatoes
- 1/2 cup cooked black beans
- 1/4 cup chopped fresh herbs (parsley, basil, chives)
- 1/4 cup crumbled goat cheese (optional)
- Salt and pepper to taste

Instructions:

1. Preheat the oven to 375°F (190°C).
2. In a bowl, combine cooked quinoa, diced tomatoes, black beans, chopped herbs, and crumbled goat cheese.
3. Stuff the bell peppers with the quinoa mixture.
4. Place stuffed peppers in a baking dish and bake for 25-30 minutes or until peppers are tender.

20.Salmon and Avocado Salad

Ingredients:

- 2 salmon fillets, grilled or baked

- 4 cups mixed salad greens

- 1 avocado, sliced

- 1/4 cup chopped red onion

- 1/4 cup chopped fresh dill

- 2 tablespoons lemon juice

- 2 tablespoons olive oil

- Salt and pepper to taste

Instructions:

1. Flake the cooked salmon into bite-sized pieces.

2. In a bowl, combine salad greens, avocado slices, chopped red onion, and flaked salmon.

3. In a separate bowl, whisk together lemon juice, olive oil, salt, and pepper to make the dressing.

4. Drizzle the dressing over the salad and toss gently to combine.

21.Berry Chia Jam

Ingredients:

- 2 cups mixed berries (strawberries, blueberries, raspberries)
- 2 tablespoons chia seeds
- 2 tablespoons honey or maple syrup

Instructions:

1. In a saucepan, heat the mixed berries over medium heat until they start to break down.

2. Mash the berries with a fork or potato masher to your desired consistency.

3. Stir in chia seeds and honey or maple syrup.

4. Continue to cook for a few more minutes until the mixture thickens.

5. Remove from heat and let the jam cool before transferring it to a jar. Store in the refrigerator.

22.Veggie and Hummus Wrap

Ingredients:

- 4 whole wheat tortillas
- 1 cup hummus (store-bought or homemade)
- 1 cup mixed sliced vegetables (bell peppers, cucumber, carrots)
- 1/2 cup baby spinach leaves
- Salt and pepper to taste

Instructions:

1. Spread a generous layer of hummus on each tortilla.
2. Layer with mixed sliced vegetables and baby spinach.
3. Season with salt and pepper, then roll up the tortillas and slice in half to serve.

23.Mango Avocado Salsa

Ingredients:

- 1 ripe mango, diced
- 1 ripe avocado, diced
- 1/4 cup diced red onion
- 1/4 cup chopped fresh cilantro
- Juice of 1 lime
- Salt and pepper to taste

Instructions:

1. In a bowl, combine diced mango, avocado, red onion, and chopped cilantro.

2. Drizzle lime juice over the mixture and gently toss.

3. Season with salt and pepper. Serve as a topping for grilled chicken, fish, or as a dip with whole-grain chips.

24.Turkey and Vegetable Stir-Fry

Ingredients:

- 1 cup cooked turkey breast, sliced

- 2 cups mixed stir-fry vegetables (snap peas, bell peppers, broccoli)

- 2 tablespoons low-sodium soy sauce

- 1 tablespoon hoisin sauce

- 1 teaspoon minced ginger

- 1 teaspoon minced garlic

- 1 tablespoon vegetable oil

Instructions:

1. Heat vegetable oil in a wok or skillet over medium-high heat.

2. Add ginger and garlic, sauté for 1-2 minutes.

3. Add sliced turkey and mixed vegetables. Cook until vegetables are tender-crisp.

4. Mix in soy sauce and hoisin sauce. Cook for an additional minute.

5. Serve over brown rice or quinoa.

25.Sweet Potato and Black Bean Bowl

Ingredients:

- 2 cups cooked quinoa

- 1 cup cooked black beans

- 1 large sweet potato, roasted and diced

- 1/2 cup salsa

- 1/4 cup chopped fresh cilantro

- Juice of 1 lime

- Salt and pepper to taste

Instructions:

1. In a bowl, combine cooked quinoa, black beans, roasted sweet potato, and salsa.

2. Drizzle lime juice over the mixture and sprinkle with chopped cilantro.

3. Season with salt and pepper. Mix well and serve.

26. Berry and Almond Smoothie

Ingredients:

- 1 cup mixed berries (strawberries, blueberries, raspberries)

- 1 banana

- 1 cup almond milk (or milk of choice)

- 2 tablespoons almond butter

- 1 tablespoon honey or maple syrup

Instructions:

1. Blend mixed berries, banana, almond milk, almond butter, and honey until smooth.

2. Pour into a glass and enjoy as a nutritious smoothie.

27.Quinoa and Roasted Vegetable Salad

Ingredients:

- 1 cup cooked quinoa

- 2 cups mixed roasted vegetables (zucchini, bell peppers, eggplant)

- 1/4 cup crumbled feta cheese

- 1/4 cup chopped fresh basil

- 2 tablespoons balsamic vinegar

- 2 tablespoons olive oil

- Salt and pepper to taste

Instructions:

1. In a bowl, combine cooked quinoa and mixed roasted vegetables.

2. Add crumbled feta cheese and chopped fresh basil.

3. In a small bowl, whisk together balsamic vinegar, olive oil, salt, and pepper to make the dressing.

4. Drizzle the dressing over the salad and toss gently to combine.

28.Apple and Walnut Chicken Salad

Ingredients:

- 2 cups cooked and shredded chicken breast
- 1 apple, diced
- 1/2 cup chopped walnuts
- 1/4 cup dried cranberries
- 1/4 cup Greek yogurt
- 1 tablespoon honey
- 1 tablespoon Dijon mustard
- Salt and pepper to taste

Instructions:

1. In a bowl, combine shredded chicken, diced apple, chopped walnuts, and dried cranberries.

2. In a separate bowl, mix Greek yogurt, honey, Dijon mustard, salt, and pepper to make the dressing.

3. Drizzle the dressing over the chicken salad and toss gently to coat.

29.Roasted Garlic and White Bean Dip

Ingredients:

- 1 can (15 oz) white beans, drained and rinsed

- 1 head of garlic

- 2 tablespoons olive oil

- Juice of 1 lemon

- 1/4 teaspoon cumin

- Salt and pepper to taste

- Fresh vegetables and whole-grain crackers for dipping

Instructions:

1. Preheat the oven to 400°F (200°C).

2. Cut the top off the head of garlic, drizzle with olive oil, and wrap in aluminum foil. Roast for about 30 minutes or until cloves are soft.

3. Squeeze the roasted garlic cloves out of the skins and into a food processor.

4. Add drained white beans, olive oil, lemon juice, cumin, salt, and pepper to the food processor. Blend until smooth.

5. Serve the dip with fresh vegetables and whole-grain crackers.

30.Greek Yogurt Parfait with Nuts and Seeds

Ingredients:

- 1 cup plain Greek yogurt

- 1/2 cup mixed nuts (almonds, walnuts, pistachios)

- 2 tablespoons mixed seeds (chia seeds, pumpkin seeds)

- 1 tablespoon honey or maple syrup

- Fresh berries for topping

Instructions:

1. In a glass or bowl, layer Greek yogurt, mixed nuts, and seeds.

2. Drizzle with honey or maple syrup and top with fresh berries.

31.Mediterranean Hummus Plate

Ingredients:

- 1 cup hummus (store-bought or homemade)

- 1 cup mixed fresh vegetables (cucumber, cherry tomatoes, bell peppers)

- 1/4 cup Kalamata olives

- 1/4 cup crumbled feta cheese

- Whole-grain pita bread or crackers for dipping

Instructions:

1. Arrange hummus in the center of a serving plate.

2. Surround the hummus with mixed fresh vegetables, Kalamata olives, and crumbled feta cheese.

3. Serve with whole-grain pita bread or crackers for dipping.

32.Lemon Herb Grilled Salmon

Ingredients:

- 2 salmon fillets

- Zest and juice of 1 lemon

- 2 tablespoons chopped fresh herbs (such as dill, parsley, thyme)

- 1 tablespoon olive oil

- Salt and pepper to taste

Instructions:

1. In a bowl, combine lemon zest, lemon juice, chopped herbs, olive oil, salt, and pepper.

2. Marinate salmon fillets in the mixture for 20-30 minutes.

3. Preheat a grill or grill pan over medium heat. Grill salmon for about 4-5 minutes per side, or until cooked through.

33.Peanut Butter Banana Smoothie

Ingredients:

- 1 banana
- 2 tablespoons peanut butter
- 1 cup milk (dairy or plant-based)
- 1 tablespoon honey or maple syrup
- 1 tablespoon flaxseeds (optional)

Instructions:

1. Blend banana, peanut butter, milk, honey or maple syrup, and flaxseeds until smooth.

2. Pour into a glass and enjoy as a satisfying smoothie.

34.Lentil and Spinach Curry

Ingredients:

- 1 cup dried green or brown lentils, rinsed and drained

- 1 onion, chopped

- 2 cloves garlic, minced

- 1 tablespoon curry powder

- 1 teaspoon ground cumin

- 1 teaspoon ground coriander

- 1 can (14 oz) diced tomatoes

- 2 cups vegetable broth

- 2 cups fresh spinach leaves

- 1 tablespoon olive oil

- Salt and pepper to taste

Instructions:

1. In a large pot, heat olive oil over medium heat. Add chopped onion and sauté until translucent.

2. Add minced garlic, curry powder, cumin, and coriander. Cook for 1-2 minutes.

3. Stir in rinsed lentils, diced tomatoes, and vegetable broth. Bring to a boil, then reduce heat and simmer for 20-25 minutes, or until lentils are tender.

4. Just before serving, stir in fresh spinach leaves and cook until wilted. Season with salt and pepper.

35.Sautéed Shrimp with Garlic and Lemon

Ingredients:

- 1 pound shrimp, peeled and deveined

- 3 cloves garlic, minced

- Zest and juice of 1 lemon

- 2 tablespoons chopped fresh parsley

- 2 tablespoons olive oil

- Salt and pepper to taste

Instructions:

1. In a bowl, combine minced garlic, lemon zest, lemon juice, chopped parsley, olive oil, salt, and pepper.

2. Marinate shrimp in the mixture for 15-20 minutes.

3. Heat a skillet over medium-high heat. Add marinated shrimp and cook for 2-3 minutes per side, or until opaque and cooked through.

36. Roasted Beet and Goat Cheese Salad

Ingredients:

- 2 medium beets, roasted and diced
- 4 cups mixed salad greens
- 1/4 cup crumbled goat cheese
- 1/4 cup chopped walnuts
- 2 tablespoons balsamic vinegar
- 2 tablespoons olive oil
- Salt and pepper to taste

Instructions:

1. In a bowl, combine diced roasted beets, mixed salad greens, crumbled goat cheese, and chopped walnuts.

2. In a separate bowl, whisk together balsamic vinegar, olive oil, salt, and pepper to make the dressing.

3. Drizzle the dressing over the salad and toss gently to combine.

37.Spaghetti Squash with Tomato Basil Sauce

Ingredients:

- 1 medium spaghetti squash

- 2 cups tomato basil sauce (store-bought or homemade)

- 1/4 cup grated Parmesan cheese

- Fresh basil leaves for garnish

- Salt and pepper to taste

Instructions:

1. Preheat the oven to 375°F (190°C).

2. Cut the spaghetti squash in half lengthwise and remove the seeds.

3. Place the halves cut-side down on a baking sheet. Bake for 30-40 minutes, or until the flesh can be easily scraped into spaghetti-like strands.

4. Use a fork to scrape the strands from the squash and transfer them to a bowl.

5. Heat the tomato basil sauce and pour it over the spaghetti squash.

6. Mix well, season with salt and pepper, and top with grated Parmesan cheese and fresh basil leaves.

38.Mushroom and Spinach Frittata

Ingredients:

- 6 eggs

- 1 cup sliced mushrooms

- 1 cup baby spinach

- 1/2 cup diced onion

- 1/4 cup shredded cheese (cheddar, mozzarella)

- 2 tablespoons olive oil

- Salt and pepper to taste

Instructions:

1. Preheat the oven to 350°F (175°C).

2. In an oven-safe skillet, heat olive oil over medium heat.

3. Add sliced mushrooms and diced onion. Sauté until mushrooms are browned and onions are translucent.

4. Add baby spinach and cook until wilted.

5. In a bowl, whisk eggs and shredded cheese together. Season with salt and pepper.

6. Pour the egg mixture over the vegetables in the skillet. Cook for a few minutes until the edges start to set.

7. Transfer the skillet to the preheated oven and bake for 15-20 minutes, or until the frittata is set and slightly golden on top.

39.Blueberry Almond Chia Pudding

Ingredients:

- 1/4 cup chia seeds

- 1 cup almond milk (or milk of choice)

- 1/2 cup fresh blueberries

- 2 tablespoons sliced almonds

- 1 tablespoon honey or maple syrup

Instructions:

1. In a bowl, combine chia seeds and almond milk. Stir well.

2. Let the mixture sit for about 15 minutes, stirring occasionally to prevent clumps.

3. Layer chia pudding, fresh blueberries, and sliced almonds in serving glasses.

4. Drizzle with honey or maple syrup before serving.

40.Tuna and White Bean Salad

Ingredients:

- 1 can (5 oz) tuna, drained and flaked
- 1 can (15 oz) white beans, drained and rinsed
- 1/2 cup diced cucumber
- 1/4 cup diced red onion
- 2 tablespoons chopped fresh parsley
- Juice of 1 lemon
- 2 tablespoons olive oil
- Salt and pepper to taste

Instructions:

1. In a bowl, combine flaked tuna, white beans, diced cucumber, diced red onion, and chopped parsley.

2. In a separate bowl, whisk together lemon juice, olive oil, salt, and pepper to make the dressing.

3. Drizzle the dressing over the tuna and white bean mixture. Toss gently to combine.

41.Chocolate Avocado Mousse

Ingredients:

- 2 ripe avocados
- 1/4 cup unsweetened cocoa powder
- 1/4 cup honey or maple syrup
- 1 teaspoon vanilla extract
- Pinch of salt
- Fresh berries for topping

Instructions:

1. In a food processor, blend ripe avocados, cocoa powder, honey or maple syrup, vanilla extract, and a pinch of salt until smooth.

2. Divide the mousse into serving glasses.

3. Refrigerate for at least 1 hour before serving.

4. Top with fresh berries before serving.

42.Lentil and Vegetable Soup

Ingredients:

- 1 cup dried green or brown lentils, rinsed and drained
- 1 carrot, diced
- 1 celery stalk, diced
- 1 onion, chopped
- 2 cloves garlic, minced
- 4 cups low-sodium vegetable broth
- 2 cups water
- 1 teaspoon dried thyme
- 1 bay leaf
- 2 tablespoons olive oil
- Salt and pepper to taste

Instructions:

1. In a large pot, heat olive oil over medium heat. Add chopped onion, diced carrot, and diced celery. Sauté until vegetables are softened.

2. Add minced garlic and cook for 1-2 minutes.

3. Stir in rinsed lentils, vegetable broth, water, dried thyme, and bay leaf.

4. Bring to a boil, then reduce heat and simmer for about 20-25 minutes, or until lentils are tender.

5. Remove the bay leaf and season with salt and pepper before serving.

43. Pesto Zucchini Noodles

Ingredients:

- 3 medium zucchinis, spiralized into noodles
- 1/4 cup basil pesto (store-bought or homemade)
- 1/4 cup cherry tomatoes, halved
- 2 tablespoons pine nuts
- Grated Parmesan cheese for garnish
- Salt and pepper to taste

Instructions:

1. In a large skillet, heat a drizzle of olive oil over medium heat.

2. Add zucchini noodles and sauté for about 2-3 minutes, or until slightly softened.

3. Stir in basil pesto and halved cherry tomatoes. Cook for another 2 minutes.

4. Toast pine nuts in a dry skillet over medium heat until lightly golden.

5. Serve the zucchini noodles topped with toasted pine nuts and grated Parmesan cheese.

44.Cauliflower Rice Stir-Fry

Ingredients:

- 1 medium head of cauliflower, riced
- 1 cup mixed stir-fry vegetables (bell peppers, carrots, peas)
- 2 tablespoons low-sodium soy sauce
- 1 tablespoon sesame oil
- 1 teaspoon minced ginger
- 1 teaspoon minced garlic
- 2 green onions, chopped
- 2 tablespoons chopped fresh cilantro
- Salt and pepper to taste

Instructions:

1. In a food processor, pulse the cauliflower until it resembles rice.

2. Heat sesame oil in a wok or skillet over medium-high heat.

3. Add minced ginger and garlic, sauté for 1-2 minutes.

4. Add mixed stir-fry vegetables and sauté until tender.

5. Push the vegetables to the side and add cauliflower rice to the wok. Cook for about 3-4 minutes, stirring occasionally.

6. Mix in soy sauce, chopped green onions, chopped cilantro, salt, and pepper. Cook for an additional 2 minutes before serving.

45.Baked Apple with Cinnamon and Walnuts

Ingredients:

- 2 apples, cored and halved
- 2 tablespoons chopped walnuts
- 1 teaspoon cinnamon
- 1 tablespoon honey or maple syrup
- Greek yogurt for topping (optional)

Instructions:

1. Preheat the oven to 350°F (175°C).
2. Place the apple halves on a baking sheet, cut side up.
3. In a small bowl, mix chopped walnuts, cinnamon, and honey or maple syrup.
4. Spoon the walnut mixture into the apple halves.
5. Bake for about 20-25 minutes, or until the apples are tender.
6. Serve with a dollop of Greek yogurt, if desired.

46.Mango Coconut Rice Pudding

Ingredients:

- 1 cup cooked white rice

- 1 mango, diced

- 1/2 cup coconut milk

- 2 tablespoons honey or maple syrup

- 1/4 teaspoon vanilla extract

- Toasted coconut flakes for garnish

Instructions:

1. In a bowl, combine cooked white rice, diced mango, coconut milk, honey or maple syrup, and vanilla extract.

2. Mix well and refrigerate for at least 30 minutes to allow flavors to meld.

3. Serve the rice pudding topped with toasted coconut flakes.

47.Creamy Pumpkin Soup

Ingredients:

- 2 cups canned pumpkin puree
- 1 cup low-sodium vegetable broth
- 1 cup coconut milk
- 1 small onion, chopped
- 2 cloves garlic, minced
- 1 teaspoon ground ginger
- 1/2 teaspoon ground nutmeg
- 2 tablespoons olive oil
- Salt and pepper to taste
- Toasted pumpkin seeds for garnish

Instructions:

1. In a pot, heat olive oil over medium heat. Add chopped onion and sauté until translucent.

2. Add minced garlic, ground ginger, and ground nutmeg. Cook for 1-2 minutes.

3. Stir in canned pumpkin puree, vegetable broth, and coconut milk.

4. Simmer for about 10-15 minutes to allow flavors to meld.

5. Use an immersion blender to blend the soup until smooth.

6. Season with salt and pepper. Serve with toasted pumpkin seeds on top.

48.Turkey Meatballs with Marinara Sauce

Ingredients:

- 1 pound ground turkey

- 1/2 cup breadcrumbs (gluten-free if needed)

- 1/4 cup grated Parmesan cheese

- 1 egg

- 2 cloves garlic, minced

- 1 teaspoon dried oregano

- Salt and pepper to taste

- 2 cups marinara sauce (store-bought or homemade)

- Chopped fresh parsley for garnish

Instructions:

1. Preheat the oven to 375°F (190°C).

2. In a bowl, combine ground turkey, breadcrumbs, grated Parmesan cheese, egg, minced garlic, dried oregano, salt, and pepper.

3. Shape the mixture into meatballs and place them on a baking sheet.

4. Bake for about 20-25 minutes, or until the meatballs are cooked through.

5. Warm the marinara sauce in a pot.

6. Serve the turkey meatballs over the marinara sauce, and garnish with chopped fresh parsley.

49.Spinach and Mushroom Omelette

Ingredients:

- 3 eggs

- 1 cup fresh baby spinach

- 1/2 cup sliced mushrooms

- 1/4 cup shredded cheese (cheddar, Swiss, or your choice)

- 1 tablespoon olive oil

- Salt and pepper to taste

Instructions:

1. In a bowl, beat the eggs and season with salt and pepper.

2. Heat olive oil in a non-stick skillet over medium heat.

3. Add sliced mushrooms and sauté until they release their moisture.

4. Add fresh baby spinach and cook until wilted.

5. Pour the beaten eggs into the skillet and swirl to evenly distribute.

6. When the eggs are almost set, sprinkle shredded cheese on one half of the omelette.

7. Fold the other half over the cheese. Cook for a minute or so until the cheese is melted.

8. Slide the omelette onto a plate and serve.

50.Herbed Brown Rice Pilaf

Ingredients:

- 1 cup cooked brown rice
- 1/4 cup chopped fresh herbs (parsley, dill, mint)
- 1/4 cup chopped dried apricots or cranberries
- 1/4 cup chopped almonds or pistachios
- 2 tablespoons olive oil
- Juice of 1 lemon
- Salt and pepper to taste

Instructions:

1. In a bowl, combine cooked brown rice, chopped fresh herbs, chopped dried apricots or cranberries, and chopped almonds or pistachios.

2. Drizzle olive oil and lemon juice over the mixture.

3. Season with salt and pepper. Mix well and serve.

51.Cucumber and Mint Infused Water

Ingredients:

- 1 cucumber, thinly sliced
- 8-10 fresh mint leaves
- Water

Instructions:

1. In a pitcher, combine cucumber slices and fresh mint leaves.

2. Fill the pitcher with water and let it sit in the refrigerator for a few hours to infuse the flavors.

3. Serve the cucumber and mint infused water chilled.

52.Coconut Quinoa Porridge

Ingredients:

- 1 cup cooked quinoa
- 1 cup coconut milk
- 1 tablespoon honey or maple syrup
- 1/4 teaspoon vanilla extract
- 1/4 cup toasted coconut flakes
- Fresh fruit (such as berries or sliced banana) for topping

Instructions:

1. In a pot, combine cooked quinoa, coconut milk, honey or maple syrup, and vanilla extract.

2. Cook over medium heat until warmed through and creamy.

3. Serve in bowls, topped with toasted coconut flakes and fresh fruit.

53.Grilled Veggie and Hummus Platter

Ingredients:

- Assorted vegetables for grilling (zucchini, eggplant, bell peppers)

- 1 cup hummus (store-bought or homemade)

- 1 tablespoon olive oil

- 1 teaspoon dried herbs (such as oregano or thyme)

- Salt and pepper to taste

Instructions:

1. Preheat a grill or grill pan over medium-high heat.

2. Toss the vegetables with olive oil, dried herbs, salt, and pepper.

3. Grill the vegetables until they are charred and tender.

4. Arrange the grilled vegetables on a platter and serve with a bowl of hummus for dipping.

54. Chickpea and Spinach Curry

Ingredients:

- 1 can (15 oz) chickpeas, drained and rinsed
- 2 cups fresh baby spinach
- 1 onion, chopped
- 2 cloves garlic, minced
- 1 tablespoon curry powder
- 1 teaspoon ground cumin
- 1 teaspoon ground coriander
- 1 can (14 oz) diced tomatoes
- 1 can (14 oz) coconut milk
- 2 tablespoons olive oil
- Salt and pepper to taste

Instructions:

1. In a large pot, heat olive oil over medium heat. Add chopped onion and sauté until translucent.

2. Add minced garlic, curry powder, cumin, and coriander. Cook for 1-2 minutes.

3. Stir in diced tomatoes and coconut milk.

4. Add chickpeas and simmer for about 15 minutes.

5. Just before serving, stir in fresh baby spinach until wilted.

6. Season with salt and pepper. Serve over brown rice or quinoa.

55.Avocado and Tomato Breakfast Toast

Ingredients:

- 2 slices whole-grain bread, toasted

- 1 ripe avocado, sliced

- 1 tomato, sliced

- 2 eggs, cooked to your preference (poached, fried, scrambled)

- Salt and pepper to taste

- Fresh herbs (such as chives or parsley) for garnish

Instructions:

1. Place the toasted bread slices on plates.

2. Top each slice with avocado slices and tomato slices.

3. Place a cooked egg on each toast.

4. Season with salt and pepper and garnish with fresh herbs.

56. Mango Ginger Smoothie

Ingredients:

- 1 ripe mango, peeled and diced
- 1 banana
- 1/2 cup Greek yogurt
- 1 teaspoon minced ginger
- 1 cup coconut water or water
- 1 tablespoon chia seeds (optional)

Instructions:

1. Blend mango, banana, Greek yogurt, minced ginger, and coconut water or water until smooth.

2. Stir in chia seeds if desired.

3. Pour into glasses and enjoy as a refreshing smoothie.

57.Broccoli and Almond Salad

Ingredients:

- 2 cups broccoli florets, blanched and chopped
- 1/4 cup sliced almonds, toasted
- 1/4 cup dried cranberries
- 2 tablespoons chopped red onion
- 2 tablespoons Greek yogurt
- 1 tablespoon lemon juice
- 1 teaspoon honey
- Salt and pepper to taste

Instructions:

1. In a bowl, combine blanched and chopped broccoli, toasted sliced almonds, dried cranberries, and chopped red onion.

2. In a separate bowl, whisk together Greek yogurt, lemon juice, honey, salt, and pepper to make the dressing.

3. Drizzle the dressing over the salad and toss gently to combine.

58.Herbed Salmon Salad

Ingredients:

- 2 cups mixed salad greens

- 1 grilled or baked salmon fillet, flaked

- 1/4 cup sliced cucumber

- 1/4 cup cherry tomatoes, halved

- 2 tablespoons chopped fresh dill or parsley

- 2 tablespoons lemon vinaigrette (olive oil, lemon juice, Dijon mustard)

- Salt and pepper to taste

Instructions:

1. In a bowl, combine mixed salad greens, flaked salmon, sliced cucumber, halved cherry tomatoes, and chopped fresh herbs.

2. Drizzle lemon vinaigrette over the salad and toss gently.

3. Season with salt and pepper. Serve as a satisfying salad.

59. Coconut Berry Chia Popsicles

Ingredients:

- 1 cup mixed berries (strawberries, blueberries, raspberries)
- 1 can (14 oz) coconut milk
- 2 tablespoons chia seeds
- 2 tablespoons honey or maple syrup

Instructions:

1. In a blender, blend mixed berries and coconut milk until smooth.

2. Stir in chia seeds and honey or maple syrup. Let the mixture sit for about 10-15 minutes to thicken.

3. Pour the mixture into popsicle molds and insert sticks.

4. Freeze for several hours or until the popsicles are firm.

60. Turmeric Cauliflower Rice Bowl

Ingredients:

- 2 cups cooked cauliflower rice
- 1 cup cooked black beans
- 1/2 cup diced bell peppers
- 1/4 cup diced red onion
- 1/4 cup chopped fresh cilantro
- 1 tablespoon olive oil
- 1 teaspoon ground turmeric
- 1/2 teaspoon ground cumin
- Juice of 1 lime
- Salt and pepper to taste

Instructions:

1. In a skillet, heat olive oil over medium heat.
2. Add diced bell peppers and red onion. Sauté until softened.
3. Stir in ground turmeric and ground cumin.
4. Add cooked cauliflower rice and black beans. Cook for a few minutes to heat through.
5. Drizzle lime juice over the mixture and season with salt and pepper.

6. Serve the turmeric cauliflower rice in bowls, topped with chopped fresh cilantro.

61. Pear and Walnut Salad with Balsamic Vinaigrette

Ingredients:

- 2 cups mixed salad greens

- 1 ripe pear, sliced

- 1/4 cup chopped walnuts, toasted

- 1/4 cup crumbled blue cheese or goat cheese

- 2 tablespoons balsamic vinaigrette (olive oil, balsamic vinegar, Dijon mustard)

- Salt and pepper to taste

Instructions:

1. In a bowl, combine mixed salad greens, sliced pear, toasted chopped walnuts, and crumbled cheese.

2. Drizzle balsamic vinaigrette over the salad and toss gently.

3. Season with salt and pepper. Serve as a refreshing salad.

62.Sweet Potato and Black Bean Tacos

Ingredients:

- 2 medium sweet potatoes, peeled and diced

- 1 can (15 oz) black beans, drained and rinsed

- 1 teaspoon chili powder

- 1/2 teaspoon ground cumin

- 1/4 teaspoon paprika

- 8 small corn tortillas

- Toppings: diced avocado, chopped cilantro, lime wedges

Instructions:

1. Preheat the oven to 400°F (200°C).

2. Toss diced sweet potatoes with a drizzle of olive oil and spread them on a baking sheet. Roast for about 20-25 minutes, or until tender and slightly caramelized.

3. In a skillet, warm the black beans and season with chili powder, ground cumin, and paprika.

4. Warm the corn tortillas in a dry skillet or microwave.

5. Assemble the tacos with roasted sweet potatoes, seasoned black beans, diced avocado, chopped cilantro, and a squeeze of lime juice.

63.Mediterranean Quinoa Salad

Ingredients:

- 2 cups cooked quinoa
- 1 cup diced cucumber
- 1 cup diced cherry tomatoes
- 1/2 cup crumbled feta cheese
- 1/4 cup chopped Kalamata olives
- 1/4 cup chopped fresh parsley
- 2 tablespoons olive oil
- Juice of 1 lemon
- Salt and pepper to taste

Instructions:

1. In a bowl, combine cooked quinoa, diced cucumber, diced cherry tomatoes, crumbled feta cheese, chopped Kalamata olives, and chopped fresh parsley.

2. In a small bowl, whisk together olive oil, lemon juice, salt, and pepper to make the dressing.

3. Drizzle the dressing over the salad and toss gently to combine.

64. Lemon Herb Baked Chicken

Ingredients:

- 4 boneless, skinless chicken breasts

- Zest and juice of 1 lemon

- 2 tablespoons chopped fresh herbs (such as rosemary, thyme, parsley)

- 2 tablespoons olive oil

- Salt and pepper to taste

Instructions:

1. Preheat the oven to 375°F (190°C).

2. In a bowl, combine lemon zest, lemon juice, chopped herbs, olive oil, salt, and pepper.

3. Place chicken breasts in a baking dish and pour the lemon herb mixture over them.

4. Bake for about 25-30 minutes, or until the chicken is cooked through and no longer pink in the center.

65.Roasted Red Pepper and Walnut Dip

Ingredients:

- 2 roasted red peppers (from a jar), drained and chopped

- 1/2 cup walnuts, toasted

- 1 clove garlic, minced

- 2 tablespoons olive oil

- 1 tablespoon lemon juice

- 1 teaspoon ground cumin

- Salt and pepper to taste

- Whole-grain pita bread or vegetable sticks for dipping

Instructions:

1. In a food processor, combine roasted red peppers, toasted walnuts, minced garlic, olive oil, lemon juice, ground cumin, salt, and pepper.

2. Blend until the dip reaches your desired consistency.

3. Serve the dip with whole-grain pita bread or vegetable sticks.

66.Chia Seed Yogurt Parfait

Ingredients:

- 1 cup Greek yogurt

- 2 tablespoons chia seeds

- 1 tablespoon honey or maple syrup

- 1/2 cup mixed berries (strawberries, blueberries, raspberries)

- 2 tablespoons granola

Instructions:

1. In a bowl, mix Greek yogurt, chia seeds, and honey or maple syrup. Let the mixture sit for about 15 minutes to allow the chia seeds to absorb the liquid.

2. Layer the chia seed yogurt mixture with mixed berries and granola in glasses or bowls.

3. Serve as a nutritious and satisfying parfait.

67.Chicken and Vegetable Stir-Fry

Ingredients:

- 1 boneless, skinless chicken breast, sliced
- 1 cup mixed stir-fry vegetables (broccoli, bell peppers, carrots)
- 2 tablespoons low-sodium soy sauce
- 1 tablespoon hoisin sauce
- 1 teaspoon minced ginger
- 1 teaspoon minced garlic
- 1 tablespoon olive oil
- Sesame seeds for garnish
- Brown rice or quinoa for serving

Instructions:

1. Heat olive oil in a wok or skillet over high heat.
2. Add sliced chicken and cook until no longer pink. Remove from the pan.
3. In the same pan, add minced ginger and garlic. Sauté for 1-2 minutes.
4. Add mixed stir-fry vegetables and cook until crisp-tender.

5. Return cooked chicken to the pan. Stir in soy sauce and hoisin sauce. Cook for a few more minutes.

6. Serve the stir-fry over brown rice or quinoa, garnished with sesame seeds.

68.Raspberry Oat Muffins

Ingredients:

- 1 cup rolled oats
- 1 cup whole wheat flour
- 1/4 cup honey or maple syrup
- 1 teaspoon baking powder
- 1/2 teaspoon baking soda
- 1/2 teaspoon cinnamon
- 1/2 cup Greek yogurt
- 1/4 cup unsweetened applesauce
- 1/4 cup milk (dairy or plant-based)
- 1 egg
- 1 cup fresh raspberries

Instructions:

1. Preheat the oven to 350°F (175°C). Line a muffin tin with paper liners.

2. In a bowl, combine rolled oats, whole wheat flour, baking powder, baking soda, and cinnamon.

3. In another bowl, whisk together honey or maple syrup, Greek yogurt, applesauce, milk, and egg.

4. Gradually add the wet ingredients to the dry ingredients, mixing until just combined.

5. Gently fold in fresh raspberries.

6. Divide the batter among the muffin cups. Bake for about 18-20 minutes, or until a toothpick inserted into the center comes out clean.

69.Greek Lentil Salad

Ingredients:

- 1 cup cooked green or brown lentils
- 1 cup diced cucumber
- 1 cup diced cherry tomatoes
- 1/2 cup diced red onion
- 1/4 cup crumbled feta cheese
- 1/4 cup chopped Kalamata olives
- 2 tablespoons chopped fresh parsley
- 2 tablespoons olive oil
- 1 tablespoon red wine vinegar
- Salt and pepper to taste

Instructions:

1. In a bowl, combine cooked lentils, diced cucumber, diced cherry tomatoes, diced red onion, crumbled feta cheese, chopped Kalamata olives, and chopped fresh parsley.

2. In a small bowl, whisk together olive oil, red wine vinegar, salt, and pepper to make the dressing.

3. Drizzle the dressing over the salad and toss gently to combine.

70.Roasted Garlic and Spinach Hummus

Ingredients:

- 1 can (15 oz) chickpeas, drained and rinsed
- 1 cup packed fresh spinach leaves
- 1/4 cup tahini
- 1/4 cup lemon juice
- 3 cloves roasted garlic
- 2 tablespoons olive oil
- 1/2 teaspoon ground cumin
- Salt and pepper to taste

Instructions:

1. In a food processor, combine chickpeas, fresh spinach, tahini, lemon juice, roasted garlic, olive oil, ground cumin, salt, and pepper.

2. Blend until the hummus is smooth and creamy. If needed, add a little water to reach the desired consistency.

3. Serve the hummus with whole-grain pita bread, vegetable sticks, or whole-wheat crackers.

71.Berry Chia Jam

Ingredients:

- 2 cups mixed berries (strawberries, blueberries, raspberries)
- 2 tablespoons chia seeds
- 1-2 tablespoons honey or maple syrup (adjust to taste)
- 1 teaspoon lemon juice

Instructions:

1. In a saucepan, combine mixed berries and cook over medium heat until they start to break down.

2. Mash the berries with a fork or potato masher to your desired consistency.

3. Stir in chia seeds, honey or maple syrup, and lemon juice.

4. Cook for an additional 5-7 minutes, stirring occasionally, until the mixture thickens.

5. Remove from heat and let the jam cool before transferring it to a jar. Refrigerate until ready to use.

72.Cauliflower and Chickpea Curry

Ingredients:

- 1 small head of cauliflower, cut into florets
- 1 can (15 oz) chickpeas, drained and rinsed
- 1 onion, chopped
- 2 cloves garlic, minced
- 1 tablespoon curry powder
- 1 teaspoon ground turmeric
- 1 teaspoon ground cumin
- 1 can (14 oz) diced tomatoes
- 1 can (14 oz) coconut milk
- 2 tablespoons olive oil
- Salt and pepper to taste
- Chopped fresh cilantro for garnish
- Brown rice or naan bread for serving

Instructions:

1. In a large pot, heat olive oil over medium heat. Add chopped onion and sauté until translucent.

2. Add minced garlic, curry powder, ground turmeric, and ground cumin. Cook for 1-2 minutes.

3. Stir in diced tomatoes and coconut milk.

4. Add cauliflower florets and chickpeas. Simmer for about 20 minutes.

5. Season with salt and pepper. Serve over brown rice or with naan bread, garnished with chopped fresh cilantro.

73.Blueberry Chia Overnight Oats

Ingredients:

- 1/2 cup rolled oats
- 1/2 cup unsweetened almond milk (or milk of choice)
- 1/2 cup fresh blueberries
- 1 tablespoon chia seeds
- 1 tablespoon honey or maple syrup
- 1/2 teaspoon vanilla extract

Instructions:

1. In a jar or container, combine rolled oats, almond milk, fresh blueberries, chia seeds, honey or maple syrup, and vanilla extract.

2. Stir well to combine, ensuring the chia seeds are evenly distributed.

3. Cover and refrigerate overnight.

4. In the morning, give the mixture a stir and enjoy your ready-to-eat breakfast.

74.Miso-Glazed Salmon

Ingredients:

- 2 salmon fillets
- 2 tablespoons white miso paste
- 1 tablespoon honey or maple syrup
- 1 tablespoon rice vinegar
- 1 teaspoon grated fresh ginger
- 1 teaspoon sesame oil
- Sliced green onions for garnish
- Cooked brown rice for serving

Instructions:

1. Preheat the oven to 400°F (200°C). Line a baking sheet with parchment paper.

2. In a bowl, whisk together white miso paste, honey or maple syrup, rice vinegar, grated ginger, and sesame oil.

3. Place the salmon fillets on the prepared baking sheet. Brush the miso mixture over the salmon.

4. Bake for about 12-15 minutes, or until the salmon is cooked to your desired doneness.

5. Serve the miso-glazed salmon over cooked brown rice, garnished with sliced green onions.

75.Roasted Beet and Goat Cheese Salad

Ingredients:

- 2 medium beets, peeled and diced

- 4 cups mixed salad greens

- 1/4 cup crumbled goat cheese

- 1/4 cup chopped walnuts, toasted

- 2 tablespoons balsamic vinaigrette (olive oil, balsamic vinegar, Dijon mustard)

- Salt and pepper to taste

Instructions:

1. Preheat the oven to 400°F (200°C). Place diced beets on a baking sheet and roast for about 20-25 minutes, or until tender.

2. In a bowl, combine mixed salad greens, roasted beets, crumbled goat cheese, and chopped toasted walnuts.

3. Drizzle balsamic vinaigrette over the salad and toss gently.

4. Season with salt and pepper. Serve as a vibrant salad.

76.Apple Cinnamon Energy Bites

Ingredients:

- 1 cup old-fashioned oats
- 1/2 cup unsweetened applesauce
- 1/4 cup almond butter
- 2 tablespoons honey or maple syrup
- 1 teaspoon ground cinnamon
- 1/2 teaspoon vanilla extract
- 1/4 cup chopped dried apples
- 1/4 cup chopped walnuts

Instructions:

1. In a bowl, combine old-fashioned oats, unsweetened applesauce, almond butter, honey or maple syrup, ground cinnamon, and vanilla extract.

2. Stir in chopped dried apples and chopped walnuts.

3. Roll the mixture into small energy bites and place them on a parchment-lined tray.

4. Refrigerate for at least 30 minutes to firm up before serving.

77.Quinoa Stuffed Bell Peppers

Ingredients:

- 4 bell peppers, tops removed and seeds removed

- 1 cup cooked quinoa

- 1 cup cooked lean ground turkey or chicken (optional)

- 1 cup diced tomatoes

- 1/2 cup black beans, drained and rinsed

- 1/4 cup diced red onion

- 1/4 cup shredded cheese (cheddar, mozzarella, or your choice)

- 1 teaspoon dried oregano

- 1 teaspoon ground cumin

- Salt and pepper to taste

Instructions:

1. Preheat the oven to 375°F (190°C).

2. In a bowl, combine cooked quinoa, cooked ground turkey or chicken (if using), diced tomatoes, black beans, diced red onion, shredded cheese, dried oregano, ground cumin, salt, and pepper.

3. Stuff the mixture into the bell peppers.

4. Place the stuffed peppers in a baking dish and bake for about 25-30 minutes, or until the peppers are tender and the filling is heated through.

78.Lemon Garlic Shrimp Pasta

Ingredients:

- 8 oz whole wheat or gluten-free spaghetti
- 1 pound large shrimp, peeled and deveined
- Zest and juice of 1 lemon
- 2 cloves garlic, minced
- 2 tablespoons olive oil
- 1/4 cup chopped fresh parsley
- Salt and pepper to taste
- Grated Parmesan cheese for garnish

Instructions:

1. Cook the pasta according to package instructions. Drain and set aside.

2. In a skillet, heat olive oil over medium heat. Add minced garlic and cook for 1-2 minutes.

3. Add shrimp to the skillet and cook until they turn pink.

4. Stir in lemon zest, lemon juice, chopped fresh parsley, salt, and pepper.

5. Toss the cooked pasta with the lemon garlic shrimp mixture.

6. Serve with a sprinkle of grated Parmesan cheese on top.

79. Herbed Quinoa Salad with Roasted Vegetables

Ingredients:

- 2 cups cooked quinoa

- 2 cups mixed roasted vegetables (zucchini, bell peppers, eggplant)

- 1/4 cup chopped fresh herbs (basil, mint, parsley)

- 1/4 cup crumbled feta cheese

- 2 tablespoons olive oil

- 1 tablespoon lemon juice

- Salt and pepper to taste

Instructions:

1. In a bowl, combine cooked quinoa, mixed roasted vegetables, chopped fresh herbs, and crumbled feta cheese.

2. In a separate bowl, whisk together olive oil, lemon juice, salt, and pepper to make the dressing.

3. Drizzle the dressing over the salad and toss gently to combine.

80.Berry Spinach Salad with Poppy Seed Dressing

Ingredients:

- 4 cups baby spinach

- 1 cup mixed berries (strawberries, blueberries, raspberries)

- 1/4 cup sliced almonds, toasted

- 1/4 cup crumbled goat cheese or feta cheese

- 2 tablespoons poppy seed dressing (olive oil, honey, Dijon mustard, poppy seeds)

- Salt and pepper to taste

Instructions:

1. In a bowl, combine baby spinach, mixed berries, toasted sliced almonds, and crumbled cheese.

2. Drizzle poppy seed dressing over the salad and toss gently.

3. Season with salt and pepper. Serve as a refreshing salad.

Please note that the information provided here is for general knowledge and should not replace professional medical advice. If you have specific concerns or questions about Brain Cancer, it's best to consult with a healthcare professional familiar with your medical history.

= THE END =

We appreciate you selecting this book! We hope your expectations were fulfilled or surpassed.

Please think about posting a review on social media if you liked our book. We value your opinion because it enables us to make improvements to our goods and services for future clients.

We want to thank you once more for your support and send our best to you.